The Diabetes Motivation Book

The Diabetes Motivation Book

Change One Thing at a Time with the

Science of Willpower

Heidi T. Beckman

Cover photograph by Antoinette Beckman
Editing by Daniel Meinen

Visit my website at www.heidibeckman.com

ISBN 978-1479215225
Library of Congress Control Number: 2012916497

Thank you to all of the individuals who have participated in my "Creative Coping with Chronic Illness" groups over the past ten years, both at the University of Wisconsin Hospital and Clinics and at Prairie View, Inc. You have taught me many important lessons about what it means to live a meaningful life with a chronic medical condition.

Table of Contents

Introduction

<u>For Whom This Book is Written</u>

Personal change is difficult. And yet, when you are diagnosed with diabetes, you are often asked to make multiple (sometimes dramatic) changes to your lifestyle. You are expected to eat the correct balance of healthy foods, to exercise regularly, to monitor your blood sugar level, and for some patients, to take medications or administer insulin. Not surprisingly, individuals with diabetes often acquire all of the necessary information about how to manage their condition, but they find themselves unable to apply it. If you have ever heard yourself say *"I know exactly what I need to do, but I can't make myself do it,"* this book is for you.

As you may have found, you can have an abundance of knowledge about healthy habits, but this does not necessarily lead to personal transformation. I have met individuals who have gone through diabetes education classes four or five times (and probably can even *teach* the class at this point!) but still do not participate in regular diabetes self-care. This situation reminds me of a quote from American author Napoleon Hill: "Knowledge is only potential power."

There is another key ingredient that must be added to your knowledge in order for you to improve your health habits and optimize your ability to cope with diabetes. That key ingredient is *motivation*. Motivation is the fuel that you need to propel yourself toward better health management. Although diabetes-specific knowledge and skills are essential first steps, motivation will ensure that you take good care of yourself well into the future.

Are you feeling a bit lacking in motivation? You're not alone. We know that changing habits for the long term is very hard. That's why 45% of people give up on their New Year's resolutions before the end of January and why many people feel that they simply cannot lose weight, quit smoking, or eat more vegetables.

Finding the motivation to cope with diabetes long-term is especially hard for several reasons. It is a condition that requires your attention on a daily basis, and you can't take a "vacation" from self-care. When you are managing diabetes, you aren't just managing what is happening in your body, but you are often managing the cognitive, emotional, and interpersonal dimensions of the disease, as well. On top of all of that, many of the complications of diabetes do not arise until well into the future (for example, vision loss, kidney problems, or nerve damage). That means you have the challenge of figuring out how to motivate yourself *today* to prevent something that won't happen until tomorrow (and therefore, is easy to ignore).

Many individuals with diabetes will acknowledge that the biggest obstacle to finding the motivation for diabetes care is their emotions. It is both normal and common to experience sadness for the losses associated with diabetes, anger or resentment, fear of future health consequences, and shame (especially if a person believes he or she is responsible for the onset of the condition). To make matters worse, symptoms associated with diabetes (like a high blood sugar level) can intensify the experience of emotional distress, and emotional distress can worsen the symptoms of diabetes.

If any of these motivational challenges sound familiar to you, this book is written for you. This is a book about *diabetes motivation* more than diabetes knowledge. It is a book about the *process of change* and finding the unique way that you can change your diabetes habits, one habit at a time.

The ideas in this book are based on well-tested willpower techniques that have been studied by behavioral scientists. These techniques have the power to transform the way you think and behave in relation to diabetes and the power to improve your self-care and health management.

If you are looking for technical details about diabetes (as you might learn in a diabetes education class), you will not find them here. However, if you are ready to learn about persistence, self-efficacy, impulse control, and other topics that are central to your diabetes motivation, this book is a good fit.

Who I Am

I am a licensed clinical psychologist who has worked in various health care settings. I am currently employed in the Department of Health Psychology at the University of Wisconsin Hospital and Clinics. I am not a medical expert; rather, I am trained to be an expert in human behavior change. As a psychologist who works with patients who have serious medical conditions, I have met hundreds of individuals who are making changes in personal health habits or lifestyle in order to optimize their ability to cope with illness.

I have written about personal change topics in newsletters, newspapers, books, and scientific journals. Writing for various publications has given me experience in accessing the literature that describes cutting-edge scientific principles, distilling that literature into something useful, and applying it to everyday problems like diabetes.

Besides my writing, a skill that I take pride in is my ability to take complex ideas out of the language of science and translate them into something relevant to everyday life. Over the past ten years, I have delivered numerous presentations on willpower and personal change to medical patients, members of the community, and professional audiences.

Perhaps most relevant to this book, I have designed and led a number of educational and psychotherapeutic groups designed to help individuals adjust to specific chronic medical conditions. Among other groups, I have offered a twelve-session group called "Change One Thing: A Group for Diabetes Self-Care." This group was designed to help people learn about the process of habit change, one lesson at a time, and then to apply each lesson to one very specific diabetes-related goal of their choosing. The group was originally intended for adults with Type 2 diabetes, but more recently, I have allowed adults with Type 1 diabetes to participate if they were interested. Because the group is more about *habit change and motivation* than it is about the specifics of diabetes, it has turned out to be a good fit for both groups of patients.

As the leader of several iterations of this group, I have had the pleasure of witnessing what happens when individuals discover how to enhance their diabetes motivation. I have seen patients become more open about their medical condition and learn how their health and their values are intimately connected. I have listened to patients report success at efforts such as eating more vegetables, exercising 10 minutes per day (when their baseline was no exercise), bringing their blood sugar meter to social gatherings (when they were too embarrassed before), reducing carbohydrate intake, introducing daily walks to the office coffee break ritual, and monitoring morning blood sugars (when the baseline was avoidance of blood sugar readings altogether).

To measure progress more objectively, I ask participants to complete a set of questionnaires at the first and last session of the group. Initial data from these questionnaires demonstrates that in general, over the course of the group, participants: (1) demonstrate an increase in self-efficacy for diabetes behaviors (meaning that their belief that they have the internal resources required to reach an important diabetes goal is strengthened); (2) increase participation in important diabetes self-care behaviors; and (3) move forward at least one stage of change with regard to a specific diabetes-related goal. Data have also shown that the hemoglobin A1c (a biological measure of how a patient's blood sugar has been over the past several months) moves in an improved direction after participation in the group. It is exciting to watch this progress.

How This Book is Different

There are many other books about diabetes management. As I've suggested, this book is different in that it is more about willpower, habit transformation, and the change process than it is about the specifics of diabetes. My intention is for you to choose one specific diabetes-related goal and work on that *one thing* over the course of the book in order to learn how *you* are uniquely motivated. Then, when you have discovered the intricacies of your diabetes motivation, you can go back and apply the same change principles to others areas of your health management.

Another thing that is different about this book is that I do not advocate any one particular theoretical model of change (for example, the cognitive-behavioral model or the motivational interviewing model). Instead, you will find that I mix together change strategies from many different areas of psychology and behavioral science. My goal is not to advocate for one theory of change or school of thought. My goal is to present the techniques that individuals with diabetes have told me they valued the most during their own personal change journeys.

How to Approach the Book

I have a special request for how you use this book. I would prefer that rather than reading it in one sitting, you absorb small bits of material and then take the time to be thoughtful and reflective about it and apply it to your own situation. To help slow down the pace of reading, there are reflection questions and activities in each unit. It is my hope that these exercises will help you develop a more potent and nuanced understanding of the complex issue of personal change. Change is certainly not a one-size-fits-all endeavor, and so it will take mental work on your end to tailor the material to your unique circumstances. You have nothing to lose by taking your time to process the issues deeply, and you might even learn something interesting about yourself, and so I recommend that you dig deep and enjoy it.

Lesson One: The Nature of Change

"For every complex problem there is an easy answer, and it is wrong."

-H. L. Mencken

"If you want to increase your success rate, double your failure rate."

-Thomas T. Watson

"The biggest room in the world is the room for improvement."

-Japanese Proverb

"A bad habit never disappears miraculously; it's an undo-it-yourself project!"

-Abigail Van Buren

In this lesson, you learn about the myths of change, and you try to establish the right mindset for doing the reflective and thoughtful work that personal change requires.

Myths About Personal Change

Myth One: Change is linear. As a person who has been diagnosed with diabetes, you have probably been asked to change many things in your life, including your eating habits, physical activity level, awareness of blood sugar levels, and perhaps your medication regimen. It is certainly easier for us to entertain the notion of change if we picture a map, consider ourselves to be at point "A," consider our end goal to be at point "B," and map out the journey as the crow flies. Ideally, the path toward a goal would be a straight line. In reality, though, change is more of a winding road where we might stop by the road and rest for a while, or even take a wrong turn or two. Tal Ben-Shahar, professor of psychology at Harvard University, describes the path toward a goal as an "irregular upward spiral… [with] numerous deviations along the way" (2009). The key point is that change takes practice, trial and error, and a repeated "coming back" to our goal.

Myth Two: Change is all-or-nothing. It is tempting to think about change as concrete: we make it to a goal, or we don't; we achieve a goal, or we fail. In reality, change is complex, and sometimes we fall in the grey area between the black and white extremes. Ultimately, though, if we create some wiggle room in our minds and accept the fact that failure and achievement can co-exist, we will persist and grow.

Myth Three: Change should happen in one try. Change is so difficult, the average self-changer has to make several attempts at a new behavior before succeeding. Change researchers Prochaska, Norcross, and DiClemente (1994) first discovered this when studying the change efforts of individuals who were addicted to substances such as alcohol, drugs, or cigarettes. They learned that most people who quit smoking report three or four serious attempts before they finally manage to kick the habit. Later, they extended their research to other types of personal change (like health behavior change) and found similar results. For instance, they found that people typically have to make a New Year's resolution for five consecutive years or more before it becomes a permanent change.

One reason that change is so difficult is because our minds are divided into independent systems that sometimes conflict. Psychologist Jonathan Haidt (2006) uses the analogy of the Elephant (the emotional side of the brain) and the Rider (the rational side of the brain). The emotional side feels pain and pleasure and likes instant gratification. The rational side is analytical and strategic and can mull over decisions with great aplomb. The Rider sits on top of the Elephant, holds the reins, and appears to be in charge most of the time. However, because he is small, he will lose to the Elephant whenever they conflict. For change to occur, there must be a goal that appeals to both the Elephant and the Rider. This does not always happen on the first change attempt.

Perhaps a good reminder to give yourself is that change is a *skill* that takes practice, practice, and more practice! Much like picking up a new musical instrument or playing a new sport, you aren't good at it on your first try. With practice, you learn which aspects of the skill come easy to you, and which aspects will require your hard work and dedication. You use this feedback to refine your approach and tailor your practice sessions. Eventually, you start to feel more confident about your ability to change. You work on one aspect of your diabetes management at a time.

Myth Four: Once you achieve initial success, it is all downhill from there. Although it is nice to experience that initial taste of pride, satisfaction, and reward when you succeed at taking the first few steps toward your goal, it does not make the rest of the journey any easier. In fact, it is pretty much guaranteed that the next set of emotions you will experience includes frustration, hardship, self-doubt, and even hopelessness. It is quite easy to feel defeated when you are trying to persist at a change effort and it feels like a struggle. Research on the "growth mindset" has shown us that there is an alternative to defeatism (Dweck, 2006). People who *know* from the beginning that "everything is hard before it is easy" and who consider struggles to be learning opportunities (rather than failures) are able to persist and to succeed in the end.

Reflection Question: Think about the personal changes you have made successfully in your life, and try to recall the details about the process of change that you went through. Did change occur as an immediate transformation or did it take practice, trial and error, and a repeated "coming back" to your goal? What emotions did you encounter along the way?

Mindset

As much as we don't like to admit it, any new endeavor is going to involve setbacks. Let's just agree to this early on and acknowledge that when we're in the middle of our change efforts, everything can look and feel like failure. As Michele Weiner-Davis, a world-renowned counselor and author, puts it: "Real change, the kind that sticks, is often three steps forward and two steps back."

If setbacks are a necessary part of the change process, then the way in which you make sense of setbacks is vital. Stanford University psychologist Carol Dweck has conducted decades of research into this issue (2006). She examines the power of mindset and how it influences our approach to goals. The conclusions she has reached teach us important lessons about how to persist as we work toward diabetes-related goals.

Dweck found that some people approach their goals with a "fixed mindset." They believe that for any given ability, we either have it or we don't, and our abilities simply reflect the way we are wired. Our fundamental qualities (like intelligence, athleticism, leadership, or health management, for example) are perceived as static. Therefore, when an opportunity comes along to strengthen a particular ability, these individuals avoid the challenge, get defensive, and see their efforts as fruitless. In the brain of a person with a fixed mindset, slip-ups simply confirm failure and verify that he or she lacks ability. In this worldview, there is really no point in attempting anything too hard, because you might just end up looking or feeling deficient in some way.

In contrast, some people approach their goals with a "growth mindset." They believe that abilities are like muscles, and they get built up with practice. When a challenge comes along, these individuals embrace the challenge, persist in the face of obstacles or setbacks, and view effort as the path to mastery. They take risks, accept feedback, and take the long-term perspective. They know that slip-ups do not mean failure or ultimate defeat. Instead, blunders mean an opportunity to learn from the mistakes and to use the feedback or criticism to reach successively higher levels of achievement.

Obviously, it is much easier to persist toward a goal when every mistake does not signal eventual failure. But how do you adopt a growth mindset if this is not the mindset that comes naturally to you? There are broad suggestions and specific ideas that might help you with this task. The broad suggestions include the following:

1. Remind yourself that everything is hard before it becomes easy.

2. Remind yourself that everything can look like failure in the middle of a change endeavor.

3. If you see something that looks like failure, remember that it is simply a sign that you are making progress and that you have taken on a worthwhile project or goal.

4. Remember that your commitment is to growth, and you can always find lessons and inspiration in your life experiences.

The specific ideas come from Carol Dweck's growth mindset workshop which she describes in her book (2006). She stresses the importance of getting specific about the "when, where, and how" with regard to something that you want to learn or a problem that you need to confront. For instance, she proposes that every morning, as you think about the day ahead of you, ask yourself: "What are the opportunities for learning and growth today? For myself? For the people around me?" Then, as you notice the opportunities for growth, form a plan to take advantage of them, and ask yourself "When, where, and how will I embark on my plan?"

If things do not go the way you want or you find yourself encountering a setback, reformulate your plan, and then ask yourself: "When, where, and how will I act on my new plan?" As you can see, there is no room in this model for judging yourself or beating yourself up when you face obstacles. Instead, there is a consistent problem-solving focus that you can come back to again and again.

Reflection Question: When you get frustrated with your diabetes change efforts, what is one reminder you can give yourself?

Homework

Decide which area of your diabetes management you would like to choose as your focus as you work through this book. It's best if you don't change goals mid-course through the book, so take your time as you choose one of the following areas:

Exercise

Healthy eating

Monitoring blood sugar levels

Taking medications as directed

Other:

Lesson Two: Stages of Change and Goal-Setting

"It's not that some people have willpower and some don't. It's that some people are ready to change and others are not."

-James Gordon

"If you don't know where you are going, you'll end up someplace else."

-Yogi Berra

"If I had six hours to chop down a tree, I'd spend the first hour sharpening the ax."

-Abraham Lincoln

Recent research in psychology has uncovered important information about the stages of change that people go through when they are trying to make a long-term change. People vary in how "ready" they are to make a change in their life. If you know something about the stage of readiness you are in, you can find the change strategies that work best. In this lesson, you will identify your stage of readiness and then design a specific goal that will focus your efforts as you work through this book.

Stages of Change

In the 1970's, change researcher James Prochaska examined many different theories of psychotherapy and identified the major themes that emerged. He was interested in determining what processes of change were common to many of the theories of psychotherapy.

Then, he and his colleagues, John Norcross and Carlo DiClemente, set out to study more than 1,000 people who were considered to be successful self-changers. They believed that the key to fostering personal change lay in the experience of the people who were able to initiate and maintain change on their own. Out of their efforts grew a six-stage model that describes the steps that people go through when making a change effort.

Stage one (precontemplation) is when a person is not particularly interested in changing and does not want to learn more about the problem. Other people may want that person to change, but that person has no intention to change in the near future. Chances are good that if you are reading this book, you are *not* in stage one with regard to your diabetes management.

Stage two (contemplation) is when a person feels pulled strongly in two different directions. On the one hand, she can name several of the potential benefits of change. On the other hand, she can name several reasons why she does not want to change or does not feel ready for change. In this stage, procrastination and feelings of ambivalence are common. Many individuals who have diabetes are familiar with the tension, discomfort, and guilt that can emerge in stage two.

Stage three (preparation) is when a person intends to take goal-consistent action soon, but she needs to get all of her ducks in a row and make a specific plan of action. As the Abraham Lincoln quote at the beginning of this lesson suggests, if you are going to cut down a tree, you need to spend a decent amount of time sharpening the ax first.

Stage four (action) is when a person has started changing his behavior and needs to work hard to keep moving forward. When the person has been successful with the new behavior for approximately six months, he moves into stage five (maintenance). In stage five, he tries to become aware of situations or conditions that might tempt him to slip back into his old behavior patterns, and he learns how to cope with these temptations in a healthy way. Finally, in stage six (termination), the individual has confidence in his new, healthy behavior and feels certain that he will not return to his old habit.

<u>Relapse</u>

Another concept that is a part of this model is that of relapse (or "recycling"), which is not one of the stages of change, but is a return from the action or maintenance stage to an earlier stage. A relapse is more than a one-time lapse or setback. It is an ongoing pattern of lapses. Typically, the person who has relapsed is flooded by thoughts and emotions that drag her down and make it challenging to get back on track. She may beat herself up mentally, thinking: "I'm a failure; I'm a loser; I'm no good."

Think about the consequences of those thoughts. If you beat yourself up, does that ultimately make you *more* task-focused and persistent or *less*? Chances are good that the negative self-talk makes you less determined and less enthusiastic about resuming your work toward your health-related goal.

We have a popular expression in our culture that if we make a mistake on a project, we are "back at square one." Prochaska, Norcross, and DiClemente, the researchers who developed the theory of the stages of change, offer a competing model for interpreting setbacks (1994). They suggest that we think about change as an *upward spiral*.

Each time you circle through a change process, you end up one level higher on the spiral. Although it may *feel* like you are back at square one, you are actually in a more elevated spot from which you can see things more clearly. At this higher perch, you are equipped with wisdom, experience, and life lessons that you didn't have when you were positioned on the level below. Using this new image, we can replace "Now I'm back at square one" with a more hopeful expression: *"Good setback, Self! You can see a lot better from this new level of the upward spiral!"* Reminding yourself of this can make a tremendous difference to your level of motivation.

Reflection Questions: Considering the area of diabetes management that you have chosen as your focus, what is your current stage of change? Is it hard for you to be honest with yourself about your true starting point for change with regard to your diabetes management? If so, what makes it hard? How can you make it "OK" to accept your current stage of change?

Change Tasks

After you determine your true starting point with regard to your diabetes management, it is time to learn how to propel yourself forward. You can now identify the "homework," self-challenges, or change tasks that will help you create movement from one stage of change to the next. It is important to know that the change tasks that you use to move from stage one to stage two are *different* from the change tasks that you use to move from stage two to stage three, and so forth. Matching your change homework to your current stage of change will help you maximize your problem solving efforts and increase the chances of success. **It might be tempting to jump into the work of the action stage, but you will not be able to sustain action unless you have completed the work of the earlier stages.**

For an individual whose starting point is the precontemplation stage of change (stage one), your primary task is to become more open-minded and less defensive about the possibility of changing a specific behavior. See if you can identify the walls that you put up to avoid thinking about change. Are you in denial about the consequences of a particular habit? Are you aware of the consequences but prone to minimizing them or explaining them away? See if you can gather information that will allow you to open up to the possibility of modifying your behavior. No need to make the decision to change at this point. You are just trying to look around, see what other people do, and see why other people think your current behavior might be problematic. Then, you can speculate why you do what you do, and pinpoint which defenses get in the way of healthier behavior. You'll know you have completed this stage when you are able to check your defenses at the door and openly consider the possibility of change.

For an individual whose starting point is the contemplation stage of change (stage two), your homework involves both "thinking tasks" and "feeling tasks." On the thinking side of things, your job is to expand your awareness of your problem behavior by monitoring how your thoughts and feelings maintain the problem. Consider completing a "decisional balance" exercise in which you create a two-by-two grid. The rows are labeled "pros" and "cons," and the columns are labeled "changing" and "not changing." When you fill in each square of the grid, take the time to consider the consequences of changing versus not changing to yourself and to others.

On the feeling side of things, your job is to get your emotions involved in your change efforts. In most change situations, you have to be able to see the problem in ways that influence your emotions, not just your thoughts. Very often, if you can't find an aspect of the problem that impacts you at the emotional level, you can't find the drive or the energy for change. The homework, then, is to imagine what the future will be like if you do NOT succeed at personal change. Attempt to paint a grim picture of the future that will shift the balance in the direction of habit modification. Key questions to ask yourself include:

- What will happen if I continue along my current path?

- What will my future look like if I do NOT make progress in this area?

- What aspects of my problem generate feelings of disappointment, disgust, or distress inside of me?

- How much power and control does my problem behavior have over me, and what positive things am I missing in my life because of it?

- What positive things might I miss out on in the future because I am refusing to change this behavior in the present?

- How do I fail myself by refusing to change this habit?

After you've painted a detailed picture of the future that focuses on the negative aspects of the problem, now shift to designing a forward-looking appraisal of how much healthier and happier life will be when you have transformed your behavior. Imagine how you will think and feel about yourself after you change. Picture yourself feeling good about yourself because your behavior is now aligned with your deepest values. You'll know you have completed this stage when you have developed a personal conviction about the value of change and the need for change. Most importantly, at this point, you have made a *decision* to pursue change. You have done something to resolve your former ambivalence and to make the "pros" of change forever outweigh the "cons."

For an individual whose starting point is the preparation stage of change (stage three), your focus will be on making a plan for the future and solidifying your commitment to change. You can start by making a list of the benefits of change and keeping it with you wherever you go. For example, if you are attempting to exercise more, write a brief list of the reasons you are exercising (the reasons that have the biggest emotional impact on you) and put copies of it in crucial places like inside your wallet and on the bathroom mirror. Your next step is to create a strong, positive image of your future self. Key questions to ask yourself include:

- After I have been successful in making this change, how will my thoughts be different? My feelings? My behavior?

- What will my new behavior free me up to achieve or become?

- In what ways will my life be enhanced once I have mastered this change?

To solidify your commitment to change, set a date that you consider to be a reasonable launch date (similar to the idea of a "quit date" for smokers). Make your commitment public. Public commitments are more powerful than private pledges because they enhance your sense of accountability, and they may help you garner social support for your efforts.

Prochaska, Norcross, and DiClemente advise that in the preparation stage, you should prepare for your change efforts in much the same way that you would prepare for a major operation or medical procedure (1994). This means putting your change plan first, and making everything else in your life second. Anticipate and prepare for the fact that your mood, your relationships with family and friends, and your daily functioning could change as you shift your energy and focus toward your change efforts.

Create a concrete plan of action. What specific steps will you take to reach your goal? What obstacles or barriers may arise that you will have to overcome? Make a list of all of the strategies that you will use to cope with the barriers to change. In addition, enlist the support of the important people in your life. Share your change plan with them and tell them specifically how they can be most helpful to you. You'll know you have completed the preparation stage when you have made a firm commitment to a detailed action plan.

Finally, for an individual whose starting point is the action stage (stage four), your primary task will be to substitute healthy responses for problem behaviors. In this stage, do anything you possibly can to set yourself up for success. Consider ways that you can "trick" yourself into doing the right thing in the moments when it will be tempting to fall back into old habits. You can probably think of several examples of this. If you're trying to eat healthier, perhaps you raid the pantry at home, throw away all of the junk food, and surround yourself with vegetables. If you're trying to exercise more, perhaps you make sure you drive by the gym on the way home from work, and you have your workout clothes ready to go in the back seat of the car.

You'll know you have completed the action stage when you have consistently executed your new behavior for approximately six months, and your new behavior now feels less effortful and more automatic.

Reflection Question: Given your current stage of readiness for change, what change strategies will work best for you (what tasks will you have to work on)?

Goal Setting

Now you are ready to create a very specific diabetes-related goal for yourself. Goal setting theory has shown that goals work because they direct your attention toward goal-relevant activities, they energize you, they lead you to persist in action over time, and they lead to the discovery and use of the right strategies for the task at hand. People who are successful at maintaining a behavior change on a long-term basis set goals with a few basic rules in mind:

- Write SMART goals (specific, measurable, achievable, realistic, and time-based)

  - Specific, challenging goals lead to better performance than nebulous goals.

  - Measurable goals allow you to gauge your progress.

- Achievable goals focus on health, are action-oriented (set "I will do" goals instead of "I will be" goals), and will fit into your life for the rest of your life.

- Realistic goals focus on ONE thing and do not include perfectionistic words such as "always," "never," "should," or "have to." Perfectionistic goals tend to be black-or-white and set you up for discouragement and failure.

- Time-based goals can be broken down into a series of steps (subgoals) that are concrete and matched to a timeline.

- Write goals that are flexible. Expect that you will revert back to your old behavior occasionally. This is a normal part of the change process.

- Write goals that are desirable and consistent with your highest values. You have to *want* it enough to make it worth it to put forth the effort.

- Physically write down your goals. This directs your attention toward your goals and starts transforming your brain in the service of your efforts.

- Write your goals in positive language. We tend to be more successful when we think of ourselves as moving *toward* something rather than moving *away* from something. (For example, consider how it feels when you think "I will eat more vegetables" versus when you think "I will not eat desserts.")

- Make your goal public. Write it on a big sign and post it on the refrigerator. Tell your friends, family members, and coworkers about your goal. Take out an ad in the newspaper and announce your goal to the world. This helps make it a matter of integrity.

- Make your goal challenging. Research suggests that we *should* shoot for the moon, as long as we have the tools, the ability, and the knowledge needed to get there.

- Make a list of the benefits associated with achieving your goal, and post this list in a place where you will see it often.

- Create a system of rewards for reaching each of the subgoals along the path to your larger goal.

- Find a way to monitor and track your progress toward your goal.

Homework

Design a specific goal for yourself that will be your focus as you work through this book. The goal should help you move forward one stage of change with respect to the specific area of diabetes management that you are working on.

Examples:

I will check my blood sugar level first thing in the morning for six out of seven days per week.

I will cook a healthy dinner for myself and my family three nights per week using recipes from my diabetes cookbook.

I will go for a walk or get on the treadmill for 10-15 minutes per day, 4-5 days per week.

I will keep a food log every day for the next two weeks so that I can bring it to my upcoming appointment with the nutritionist.

I will put together an exercise action plan and ask for the specific kind of social support I need before I reach my launch date of July 6.

Lesson Three: Develop the Identity of a Changer

"The value of identity, of course, is that so often with it comes purpose."

-Richard R. Grant

In this lesson, you will learn how to make your change effort part of your overall sense of self.

Change as a Matter of Identity

In one of the groups that I lead at my workplace, I give group members an "official changer card" that they can carry with them to remind them of their change efforts. Research evidence points to the idea that if you make your change effort a bigger part of your identity, you will be more likely to make the kinds of decisions that will support your end goal. At the same time, any change effort that violates your identity will be doomed to eventual failure.

I met someone recently who gave me a fantastic example of this. He said that he used to show up late for everything—meetings, events, social gatherings, and so on. He told me that he hit a turning point rather abruptly one day. Thinking to himself, "That's it! I'm not going to be a late person anymore," he transformed his self-image into that of a person who shows up on time or even early. After he started defining himself in a new way, he was never late again.

Reflection Question (adapted from Heath & Heath, 2010): Do you agree with this statement: "I aspire to be the kind of person who would make this change."

If yes, then your identity will support your change efforts.

If no, do you need to change your goal? Or do you need to convince yourself to aspire to a different self-image or identity? Remember, you can cultivate a new identity. Identities grow from small beginnings.

Self-As-Doer

Researchers Linda Houser-Marko and Kennon Sheldon have started a line of research on the "self-as-doer" construct (2006). There is good evidence that if you think of yourself as the "doer" of an action, you are more likely to persist at that task, even when obstacles emerge. For example, if I think of myself as a "runner," I am more likely to go out and run every morning, even when storm clouds gather on the horizon or when my shoes don't fit me quite right.

Here are some diabetes-related examples:

"I am a healthy eater."

"I am a stair-climber."

"I am a blood sugar level checker."

Reflection Question: How can you think of yourself as a "doer" of healthy behaviors?

Complete this statement in support of your goal:

"I am a _____."

<u>Homework</u>

Write your identity statement on several post-it notes, and stick the post-it notes in obvious places where you will see them over the next seven days: on your refrigerator, your steering wheel, your computer monitor, your wallet. Each time you encounter a sticky note, read the statement and really try to feel the sense of pride and accomplishment that accompanies the realization that this is a part of your identity.

Lesson Four: Align Your Change With Your Values

"None of us will ever accomplish anything excellent or commanding except when he listens to this whisper which is heard by him alone."

-Ralph Waldo Emerson

If you have a deep understanding of what is most important to you, then you will be able to design meaningful goals. Any serious change journey includes a consideration of values. In this lesson, you will examine your values and consider how they relate to your diabetes management.

Values Versus Goals

Values and goals are two very different things. Think of your values as the compass that points you in the direction you wish to go in life. Your goals, then, are the practical, achievable objectives that move you in your valued direction. As Dahl and Lundgren explain, "Values are lifelong paths that vitalize your life by giving it direction and meaning. You live your values all your life; they never end. Goals, on the other hand, have an end point" (2006).

Values reflect a range of concepts, principles, and beliefs that are important to you and that you hold dear. Therefore, when your behaviors are not in line with your deepest-held values, this will create internal conflict and discomfort. To make sure you have energy and persistence in your change efforts, *set goals that are consistent with your highest values.*

One of the biggest reasons why people fail to accomplish goals is because it does not fit in with what is most important to them. Here is a list of the kinds of things that people can value. Read through the list and circle the ones that are most important to you. Add any of your values that are missing from the list.

Abundance	Helpfulness
Achievement	Hope
Adventure	Independence
Attractiveness	Influence
Beauty	Knowledge
Comfort	Leisure
Confidence	Loyalty
Connection with others	Moderation
Creativity	Organization
Excellence	Peace of mind
Family	Play
Flexibility	Popularity
Freedom	Power
Friends	Responsibility
Fulfillment	Risk
Fun	Security
Generosity	Service
Growth	Simplicity
Happiness	Solitude
Harmony	Spirituality
Health	Stability

Strength   World peace

Tradition   Other:

From the values you selected, choose your top five. Then prioritize them from most important to least important. List them here:

Sometimes our behaviors do not match with what we value most in life. Think about the area of your diabetes management that you are working on as you read this book. Can you think of times when your behavior in this area has conflicted with or has been inconsistent with your values? For example, perhaps you decided that family is one of your core values, but you are not taking care of your health in a way that allows you to be fully present and available to your family. Or perhaps you have decided that stability and peace of mind are core values, but you are allowing your blood sugar levels to range widely. In these examples, your behavior is inconsistent with your values. Now consider this: What do you need to do to bring your health behavior into alignment with your values? Also, does the diabetes goal that you have chosen fit with your highest priorities?

While on the topic of values, let's consider a different, somewhat tricky issue. One of the reasons why changing a behavior can be so difficult is that we may really value that behavior under a different name. For example, I may consider myself to have a problem with overeating, and I may pledge to modify this habit once and for all. However, maybe somewhere deep inside my brain, overeating is equated with comfort, abundance, recreation, celebration, or social connectedness, and these are values with which I am not willing to part. To change my overeating, then, I may need to refine my understanding of my behavior. As Ben-Shahar writes, "To be able to change, we need a nuanced understanding of what exactly it is that we want to get rid of and what we want to keep" (2009). Your task is to unpackage (or "unbundle") the concept of overeating and ask yourself several questions:

- What does overeating mean to me?

- Is there a different way for me to achieve these gains in my life without risking my health? (For example, if I tend to overeat at celebratory gatherings, is there a tactful way for me to bring food to these gatherings that will not violate my nutritional plan?)

- What elements of overeating can I afford to keep? (For example, can I work with my nutritionist to design a plan that allows for certain "treats" under certain conditions?)

- What elements of overeating do I want to get rid of because they exact too much of a cost?

These questions should get you started in designing a goal that is truly desirable to you, without the risk of losing something else that you value.

Homework

Sometimes our behaviors do not match with what we value most in life. In the past, what are the ways that your health behavior has had a negative impact on each of your core values?

Which of your values provide motivation for you to change your health behavior?

Is the goal that you set for yourself consistent with your highest values?

Over the course of the upcoming week, notice any diabetes-related or self-care behaviors that you engage in that **do not match with or support your values.**

Over the course of the upcoming week, notice any diabetes-related or self-care behaviors that you engage in that **support and are consistent with your values.**

What do you need to do to bring your self-care into alignment with your values?

Lesson Five: Keep Up Your Energy Level

"Big problems are rarely solved with commensurately big solutions. Instead, they are most often solved by a sequence of small solutions."

-Chip Heath and Dan Heath

In this lesson, you will learn why it can sometimes be exhausting to change something about your behavior, like starting to count carbohydrates or monitor your blood sugar on a regular basis. Then, you will read about three potential ways to keep up your energy level during the change process.

Regulatory Depletion

Unfortunately, self-control is a limited, exhaustible resource. Picture yourself carrying a "bucket of self-control" throughout the day. When you wake up in the morning (provided that you got sufficient, restful sleep), your bucket is full. You feel abundant strength and energy to engage in tasks that require you to supervise yourself closely, to focus your attention, to be careful with your behavior, to inhibit your impulses, and to persist in the face of emotional obstacles. (Think about how many of these tasks are central to diabetes management.)

When you walk through your day, then, you slowly use up the supply of self-control in your bucket. When your bucket approaches empty, it becomes much harder to think creatively in the face of challenges. You do not feel like you have the energy to transform bad habits or avoid temptation.

There are many different tasks that use up the supply of self-control in the bucket. The bucket drains whenever we resist temptation, hold back distressing emotions, suppress forbidden thoughts, and try to make a choice from an overabundance of options (Baumeister et al., 1998). Included in that list are many of the situations that we may encounter on a daily basis, such as resisting donuts, making sure we don't speed on the way home from work, and managing the impression that we make on other people.

What is the end result of all of this restraint, suppression, and self-supervision? According to the research literature, the consequence for us is diminished physical and cognitive stamina. We also end up with less flexibility and creativity along with an inability to persist in the face of failure. The official name for this is *regulatory depletion. It means that if we use up much of our supply of self-control on one task, we have limited self-control available to use on the next task.* For example, if research participants work hard to suppress their thoughts or feelings during an initial task, they have less stamina available to them to control their bodies or minds on a subsequent task, even if it is a completely different task that is perceived to be unrelated.

Imagine how this applies to diabetes care. If you use up most of your supply of self-control during the workday by suppressing the mean thoughts you are having about a coworker, resisting the candy dish that sits next to the copy machine, and/or overriding your true feelings in the service of your customers or clients, how would you have enough self-control left when you get home? Many people believe they make unhealthy food choices in the evening because they are physically tired from the workday. This theory suggests that they are making poor choices because are suffering from regulatory depletion, not physical exhaustion.

The take-home message, as stated by Chip and Dan Heath (2010), is this: "What looks like laziness is often exhaustion. Change wears people out—even well-intentioned people will simply run out of fuel."

Solution One: Find the "Exceptions"—What is Working Well?

One possible solution is to look for the things that are working well already, and then try to replicate these conditions.

The key question is "What is working, and how can I do more of it?"

Think about the area of your diabetes care that you are attempting to change.

Now think about the times in the **past** when you were coming close (or closer) to taking good care of yourself in that domain. What were you doing differently then? What encouraging, optimistic, or helpful thoughts were you thinking back then?

Now think about the times in the **present** when you come close (or closer) to your goal. What is different during those times? What are you doing, thinking, and feeling during those times?

Solution Two: Identify the Specific Behavior You Want to See in a Tough Moment

Sometimes when we think about the "big picture" and what needs to change, we get lost in all of the possibilities. As a result, we end up following the status quo instead of following through with a personal change.

We need simple rules to fall back on at these times. You can create these rules by identifying the specific behaviors you want to see in a tough moment. Make your rules behavioral, specific, and concrete. Authors Chip and Dan Heath call this "scripting the critical moves" (2010). They remind us that clarity will help dissolve resistance.

The key question is "What are the critical actions that I want to see myself carry out even when I feel too overwhelmed to make good progress toward my goal?"

Complete this sentence: If I can do nothing else, I will at least

_____.

Examples:

If I can do nothing else, I will at least carry my meter with me at all times.

If I can do nothing else, I will at least walk into the gym, change into my gym clothes, do five minutes of exercise, and then evaluate how I feel about continuing or not.

Solution Three: Create a Picture of What is Possible

According to the Heath brothers, "Change is easier when you know where you're going and why it's worth it" (2010). They suggest that if we can point ourselves toward an attractive destination, we will start figuring out how to get there.

They recommend designing something called a "destination postcard," which is a vivid picture from the near-term future that shows what could be possible.

The key question is "Where am I headed in the end? What's my destination?"

If you were to tape a postcard to your refrigerator that represents your end goal, what image would it have?

If you were to design a t-shirt or bumper sticker that epitomizes your end goal, what would it say?

<u>Homework</u>

Now back up your destination postcard with a detailed motivational plan. Complete the following worksheet (adapted from Wiseman, 2009).

My Motivational Plan

My overall goal is to…

Break your goal into five smaller steps. For each step, consider:

>The sub-goal is...

>I believe that I can achieve this goal because...

>To achieve this sub-goal, I will...

>This will be achieved by the following date...

>My reward for achieving this will be...

What are three benefits of achieving my overall goal? List three benefits associated with your desired future.

Whom will I tell about my goal and sub-goals?

Lesson Six: Use Your Emotions in Your Favor

"The truth is that our finest moments are most likely to occur when we are feeling deeply uncomfortable, unhappy, or unfulfilled. For it is only in such moments, propelled by our discomfort, that we are likely to step out of our ruts and start searching for different ways or truer answers."

-M. Scott Peck

"Human behavior flows from three main sources: desire, emotion, and knowledge."

-Plato

Very often, when we face a long road toward a health-related goal and we see no signs of progress or reassurance, we slow down or stop. In this lesson, you will learn two ways to harness your emotions to provide the energy and drive to keep working toward your goal.

Solution One: Find the Feeling Behind the Need for Change

In most change situations, you have to be able to see the problem or solution in ways that influence your *emotions*, not just your thoughts. As you learned when you read about the contemplation stage of change, you have to find something that hits you at the emotional level, such as (1) a disturbing look at the problem, (2) a hopeful glance at the solution, or (3) discomfort when you recognize the distance between where you *are* and where you *wish to be*.

The key question is "What will happen if you continue along your current path?"

Write your story of the future, or draw a picture of the future, assuming that you do NOT make progress toward your goal. Make your story as rich and detailed as possible.

At this point, you may be wondering if you need to create negative emotions (fear, anxiety, terror, doom) or positive emotions (hope, joy, pride, gratitude) in order to motivate yourself. After reviewing the literature, Chip Heath and Dan Heath (2010) concluded that if you need quick and specific action toward your goal, it might be most helpful to generate negative emotions. However, if you want to broaden your creativity, ingenuity, and flexibility in your approach to your goal, positive emotions will be most effective.

In general, with long-range diabetes goals that will require you to constantly refine your approach, you may benefit most from the open mind and broadened view generated by positive emotions. However, if your current stage of change is the contemplation stage, you may get a motivation boost from the discomfort of negative emotions, as well.

Solution Two: Find Some Way to Engineer Small Successes Early On

I have seen no better movie about personal change efforts than The King's Speech, which won the Academy Award for "Best Picture" in 2011 (produced by Canning, Sherman, & Unwin, 2010). The movie is the story of Albert, the Duke of York, who suddenly became King George VI of the United Kingdom and was forced to confront his life-long struggle with stuttering. His speech therapist, Lionel Logue, employed a number of creative strategies to help the king improve his speech and, perhaps more importantly, overcome fear. In the movie, the king made a transformation from a hesitant, self-doubting, temperamental man to a capable and more confident king.

In the movie, the speech therapist who worked with the king made an important observation early in their work together. He noticed that the king felt demoralized and hopeless with regard to the possibility of correcting his speech. The king repeated dejected utterances such as "I can't" and "No one can fix it." The speech therapist was astute enough to realize that the king needed to experience an "early success" in order to reverse the feelings of hopelessness and strengthen his commitment to treatment. Therefore, he engineered a situation in which the king could hear a recording of himself reading a passage aloud with no stuttering. Sure enough, when the king played the recording, it prompted his decision to return to the speech therapist's office for further treatment, even though he had previously given up and stormed out.

This is a good illustration of the importance of mastering a small step or engineering an "early win." When we experience a sense of mastery over a small step, our feelings of hopelessness are converted into reassurance. We build confidence that we can, indeed, make forward progress toward our goal because after all, we have already conquered part of it. Many people find it more motivating to be partly finished with a longer journey than to be at the starting line of a shorter one. If we design situations in which we can achieve early success (even if they are small steps), this will counteract feelings of doubt, defeat, or discouragement.

Psychologist Karl Weick describes the purpose of a small win this way: "A small win reduces importance ('this is no big deal'), reduces demands ('that's all that needs to be done'), and raises perceived skill levels ('I can do at least that')" (1984). These three factors combine to help us replace feelings of dread with confidence and hope.

In the context of your health management, how can you engineer a small success early on in order to strengthen your belief in yourself and your personal resources? If your goal is to choose healthier foods for your evening meal, what is one small step you can take today? Can you begin by researching recipes, planning your next trip to the grocery store, or having a collaborative discussion with the designated household cook? It that is too big of a leap, can you begin by asking friends, family members, or coworkers what success strategies they have found to help them eat healthy foods in the evening?

Complete this sentence: For me, a goal that is within immediate reach is _____.

Examples:

I will find my blood sugar meter.

I will take a tour of the local health club.

I will start making a list of questions that I wish to ask my nutritionist.

It is OK if your small wins seem trivial. Big changes come from a series of small changes. In this way you can turn a sense of dread into confidence and pride.

Homework

Identify what feeling you will foster to inspire you to work toward your diabetes goal. Also, design a couple of "small wins" that are meaningful and within immediate reach, and write them in on your calendar for the next week. Check them off of your calendar each day as you make them happen.

Lesson Seven: Use Your Body in Your Favor

"Our own physical body possesses a wisdom which we who inhabit the body lack."

-Henry Miller

"There is a wisdom in the body that is older and more reliable than clocks and calendars."

-John Harold Johnson

———⧓———

This lesson may seem to pose a dilemma at first glance. How can you use your body in support of your health-related goal when very often, in the course of day-to-day diabetes management, you feel like you are fighting with your body? Read on to find out how some very simple, physiological self-care strategies can actually *reduce* the willpower struggle by influencing the level of impulse control that is available to you.

Biological Response Patterns

You have probably heard about (and no doubt, experienced more than one time!) the body's fight-or-flight response. Sometimes referred to as the adrenaline response, this is the set of changes that occurs in the body when you perceive a threat, like a hungry tiger chasing you down the street, a driver veering into your lane of traffic, or a coworker uttering an insult. In these situations, the brain sets off an alarm signal that tells the rest of the body to get ready to either fight the situation somehow or to run from it. During the fight-or-flight response, the body diverts energy *away* from the area of the brain that is responsible for planning, judgment, and deliberation and *toward* the large muscle groups of the body that will help you fight or run. No doubt, it's a useful physiological response mechanism to have. However, it is not very conducive to careful decision-making.

Dr. Suzanne Segerstrom, a psychologist at the University of Kentucky, has identified and named an entirely different biological response, one that supports the thinking resources we so desperately need when we are caught in a willpower struggle. She calls it the "pause-and-plan response" and suggests that is a set of changes that occurs in the body when we need to suspend our impulses on a temporary basis and focus on our long-term goals (Segerstrom & Solberg Nes, 2007). It all starts with our brains perceiving one of two kinds of internal conflict: (1) we want to do something but know that we shouldn't, like eat the whole carton of ice cream; or (2) we know we should do something but really don't want to, like go to the gym. When the pause-and-plan response kicks in, the brain diverts energy *away* from the body (and lowers heart rate, breathing rate, and blood pressure) and *toward* the area of the brain that helps us engage in flexible, thoughtful action. This is what helps us stay calm in the face of temptation and focus on our long-term goals instead of our immediate impulses.

The important question, then, is this: How do we increase the chances that our brains and bodies will be able to shift into the pause-and-plan response? The simplest way to support the physiology of willpower and to train yourself to get better at self-control is through slow, relaxed, even breathing, preferably at a rate of four to six breaths per minute. This may take some practice at first, but if you simply practice a few minutes at a time and sprinkle the practice throughout your day, you will find yourself able to do this effectively after a few trials.

<u>Mindfulness of Breath Exercises</u>

Here are some examples of simple ways to shift your attention toward your breath and to slow down the pace of your breathing:

- Shift your attention to the point at the tip of the nose, in-between the two nostrils. Notice the flow of air coming in when you inhale and going out as you exhale. You may even notice a small temperature difference at the tip of your nose: the air that flows in is slightly cool, while the air that flows out is slightly warm.

- Or, shift your attention to the center of your abdomen. Notice the rising of the belly on the inhale and the falling of the belly on the exhale.

- Practice counting slowly to "4" when you inhale and counting to "5" or "6" when you exhale. When your exhale is longer than your inhale, this will slow down the overall pace of your breathing.

- Try breathing in through your nose and out through your mouth, completing ten cycles of breath, striving to make each in/out cycle slightly longer than the previous one.

Remember, regular practice is important. Through regular practice, you are training yourself to get better at a wide range of self-control skills, such as focusing your attention, decreasing your reactivity to your impulses, and increasing your self-awareness.

<u>Other Self-Care Strategies</u>

While mindful breathing is probably the number one physiological self-care strategy you can use to strengthen your willpower, there are other important strategies that help with this, as well. For example, simple things like getting a good night's sleep, engaging in five-minute doses of exercise, and getting a breath of fresh air (outside) can go a long way to strengthen your self-control. Relaxation strategies such as the body scan technique or peaceful imagery may help you shore up your willpower reserves. In the interpersonal domain, spending quality time with supportive, healthy people can boost your confidence and strengthen your ability to resist temptation.

Reflection Question: What is one self-care activity I can work into my daily routine? I will remind myself that this will ultimately make more self-control available to me when I face willpower challenges.

Homework

Can you spare five minutes? Challenge yourself to choose one five-minute self-care activity and work it into your schedule every day for the next seven days. It might be something as simple as five minutes of deep breathing when you are waiting for your coffee, waiting for photocopies, or waiting in line at the grocery store!

Lesson Eight: Use Your Environment in Your Favor

"The block of granite which was an obstacle in the pathway of the weak becomes a stepping-stone in the pathway of the strong."

-Thomas Carlyle

Another way to make progress toward your goal is to find ways to make the right behaviors easier and the wrong behaviors harder (or even impossible). In this lesson, you will learn ways to tweak the environment to increase the chances that you will engage in goal-directed behavior.

Change the Environment

When you're working on a personal challenge like eating healthier or exercising more, what does it take to "trick" yourself into doing the right thing? How can you change the environment in order to set yourself up for success? Can you change the foods that you have available in your household? Obtain multiple meters and put them in several places around your home and workplace? Put your medications next to your toothbrush?

My all-time favorite example of tweaking the environment came from a participant in my diabetes group. Her goal involved increasing her overall level of physical activity. She decided to move her stationary bicycle into the center of her living room, directly in front of the television. In this way, the bike would block her view of the TV screen if she were sitting anywhere else in the room. If she wanted to watch TV, she *had* to sit on the bike. And if she was sitting on the bike, well...she might as well do some pedaling.

Chip Heath and Dan Heath refer to this technique as "tweaking the environment" or "shaping the path" (2010). Richard Thaler and Cass Sunstein call this a "nudge"—setting up the options to alter our behavior in a particular (favorable) way (2008).

From a psychology standpoint, it makes great sense because our calm, cool, rational side is easily overwhelmed by the emotions of the moment. So whatever we can do to make the desired behaviors easier and the undesired behaviors more difficult, we should do it.

Reflection Question: How can I set up my environment to make the right behaviors easier and the wrong behaviors harder (or even impossible)?

Build Habits

According to Chip and Dan Heath, *action triggers* are conditions that you can set up that will increase the chances that you engage in your desired behavior when you encounter a certain environmental reminder or trigger. The basic formula for an action trigger is: "When X occurs, Y will occur." Here are some diabetes-related examples:

- When I go out to get my morning newspaper, I will take a short walk.

- When I sit down at a table in the restaurant, I will put my meter out on the table as a reminder to myself.

- When I brush my teeth, I will take my medication.

According to the Heath brothers, action triggers are helpful because they "preload the decision;" that is, they allow you to make the right decision before you arrive at the moment of temptation, and there is no conscious deliberation necessary. They essentially protect your goals from distractions and competing goals by passing the control of your behavior onto the environment.

Reflection Question: What action trigger can I set up that will protect my diabetes-related goal from tempting distractions or bad habits?

Lesson Nine: Exercise Your Self-Control Muscle

"Grant us a brief delay; impulse in everything is but a worthless servant."

–Caecilius Statius

"I generally avoid temptation unless I can't resist it."

–Mae West

In this lesson, you learn that you can strengthen your self-control with practice, much like your muscles can be built up through regular strength training.

Importance of Self-Discipline

We know that people vary in their ability to choose successfully between conflicting desires and impulses. We also know that the road to success often requires self-control (also referred to as self-discipline), or choosing long-term gain over short-term pleasure: resisting a decadent piece of cheesecake in the service of losing weight, enduring the hardship of homework in order to achieve good grades, or passing up the unplanned purchases to stick to the household budget.

Research on self-discipline has shown that it is a crucial factor in predicting people's future success. It forecasts who will be able to do what is required of them (and therefore achieve important goals) versus who will wander down the path of temptation.

Researcher Angela Duckworth and her colleagues use the term "grit" to refer to self-discipline (2007). According to Duckworth, if a person is "gritty," he or she is not thrown off course by disappointment, failure, adversity, boredom, or plateaus in progress. While an impulsive person might use these elements as an excuse to give up, the gritty individual chooses to keep working strenuously toward challenges.

How Do I Strengthen My Self-Control?

There is a program of exercise that is unlikely to show up as a class at your gym, and yet it has the power to transform your entire life: self-control training. Exercising your impulse control muscle can literally transform the landscape of your brain and train your mind to be better at self-observation, to pause before acting impulsively, and to choose the more difficult path when it serves your larger goals.

Imagine how these skills could benefit your self-care and health management. If you strengthen your impulse control, it would be so much easier to choose a smaller portion size when you are tempted to overeat, to be patient with a new exercise program instead of reacting to bumps in the road, and to check your blood sugar consistently instead of being lured into the immediate pleasures of the moment.

Just as a gym-based exercise program allows us to meet physical challenges with greater ease, a willpower workout allows us to meet physical, mental, emotional, environmental, and societal challenges with greater ease (see the work of psychologist Roy Baumeister).

How do you do it? Psychologist Kelly McGonigal, in her recent book *The Willpower Instinct* (2011), reviews three categories of self-control training:

1. *Add new habits*: Pick one thing to do every day just for the practice of building up a habit. Dr. McGonigal suggests tasks such as finding one thing in your house that needs to be

thrown away, calling a specific person, or focusing on your breath for five minutes.

2. *Avoid old habits*: Pick one thing to not do every day simply for the practice of noticing your old habits and then choosing a more difficult path. For example, avoid crossing your legs when you sit, avoid swearing, substitute the word "yes" for "yeah," or use your nondominant hand for eating.

3. *Keep track of something*: Choose an activity that you don't ordinarily monitor and keep a formal record of it. For example, track how much time you spend online, how much time you watch television, or how many times you go up and down the stairs at your house.

These may seem like trivial changes, but research shows that these practices are a powerful way to help the brain grow stronger at self-control. They train you to notice your behavior, pause before acting, and choose to do the more difficult thing. And just think: You don't even have to buy spandex to join this exercise revolution!

Reflection Questions: What is an area of my life in which I have shown great self-discipline? How can I access this skill and apply it to my diabetes management efforts?

Homework

Choose one willpower exercise to practice every day for the next seven days. Notice how you feel about yourself each time you accomplish this small challenge.

Lesson Ten: Manage Difficult Emotions

"Your emotions follow your thoughts, just as surely as baby ducks follow their mother. But the fact that baby ducks follow faithfully along doesn't prove that the mother knows where she is going!"

-David Burns

"We either make ourselves miserable or we make ourselves strong. The amount of work is the same."

-Carlos Castaneda

It is common for emotions such as depression, anger, fear, and guilt to emerge when you are working hard on a personal change effort. In this lesson, you will discover how to walk alongside these emotions *and* keep doing the things you need to do to improve your health.

When Emotions Are Problematic

When you are working hard to change something about your health behavior, any and all emotions are par for the course. Remember that these emotions are normal, healthy, human, and understandable. Emotions tend to come and go like waves in the ocean. When they emerge, they give us important cues about a situation and our relationship to it. We can use these cues to decide upon an appropriate reaction or response.

When do emotions become problematic? Emotions are considered to be problematic when they are so negative or inflexible that they get in the way of our daily functioning or they make it very difficult for us to adapt to the circumstances in which we find ourselves. For example, when emotions interfere with our self-care, they deserve extra attention.

Emotions are also considered to be problematic if we get so rigidly entrenched inside a particular feeling, we apply it to every aspect of our experience. For instance, if you get locked into an anger pattern and you become angry about diabetes, angry at the people who are trying to help you with your diabetes, and angry at yourself for your health dilemma, then the emotion definitely warrants a closer look.

When faced with a problematic emotion, it is important not to push it away, pretend it isn't there, or stuff it beneath the surface of your consciousness. Tucking emotions away just leads to more distress in the long run. Start by being aware of the feeling, acknowledging that it is there, and being open to what it is trying to tell you. The more you can allow yourself to approach the feeling with an attitude of openness and curiosity (rather than judgment and self-disparagement), the less overwhelming it will become.

Depression in Diabetes

The reality of living with diabetes is that it is a life-long challenge to a person's intellectual, physical, and emotional coping skills. Diabetes is a difficult, demanding, and often stressful condition. Feelings of uncertainty, loss, and sadness in people with diabetes are common and normal and need to be acknowledged.

When feelings of sadness persist and when they are accompanied by a number of other cognitive, emotional, and physiological symptoms (like fatigue, diminished motivation, diminished concentration, and feelings of hopelessness or worthlessness), we call it a depressive syndrome or clinical depression. If we look at research findings about the prevalence of depression in the population of adults who have diabetes, we find this:

- Depression is more prevalent in individuals with diabetes than in the general population.

- The prevalence of depression in the population of individuals with diabetes is believed to be 14-15%, which is at least three times the prevalence of major depressive disorder found in the general adult population.

- There are two possible reasons why individuals with diabetes are more prone to depression:

- They are dealing with the stress of a chronic condition.

- They have experienced metabolic changes (that is, the disease alters your physiology in some ways).

Here is the problem: Depression has a negative impact on your level of energy, focus, and motivation, and it has the potential to drive supportive people away. If you do not have your typical level of energy, focus, and motivation, how are you going to be able to engage in good diabetes self-care?

Coping With Depression

If you suspect you have clinical depression, the most important thing you can do is talk with a mental health professional, your primary care physician, or another health provider who is knowledgeable about the condition. When you are depressed, it is hard to imagine that you can ever feel better again. Just remember that this is one of the "tricks" that depression plays on your brain: It makes you believe that the future will be just as bad as, or worse than, the present. Know that depression is a treatable condition and that many, many people perceive benefit from psychotherapy, medications, or a combination of the two treatments.

After you have told a health care provider about your depression, here are some other things you can do that may help you cope with your depression:

- Teach yourself that bad feelings are not intolerable or scary. You can have your bad feelings and still do the things you need to do to take care of yourself.

- Reduce your alcohol intake or stop drinking altogether. Alcohol is a depressant and can maintain or worsen depressive symptoms.

- Continue your daily activities. Maintaining structure in your day is one of the most helpful things you can do for yourself.

- Visit with friends, family, and neighbors. When you become depressed, your world starts to get smaller and you begin isolating yourself from the important people in your life. The antidote to depression is reaching out, even though you may not feel like doing this at first.

- Join a group.

- Volunteer.

- Make plans and carry them out.

- Take a vacation.

- Exercise. Many research findings have shown that moderate physical activity can be just as effective as antidepressant medication in helping some people manage mild depressive symptoms.

- Use positive self-talk.

- Focus on your future goals.

- Focus on what you are thankful for.

Coping With Anger

Anger often occurs secondary to a primary emotion. If you look closer at your anger, you may find that frustration, hurt, or fear of loss are hiding behind an angry feeling. Many people with diabetes express anger at the perceived unfairness that they have to live with this condition when other people around them do not. They express anger at themselves for their belief that they may have gotten themselves into this health predicament due to years of neglecting their self-care. Or, they express anger at their medical providers for getting on their case about high blood sugar values. Some individuals with diabetes feel that their medical providers do not truly understand how difficult it is to manage the many facets of the condition, and this leads to feelings of anger and resentment.

If we hold on to anger, rather than using it as an impetus for constructive action, it can be destructive to us over time. Buddha is believed to have said, "Holding on to anger is like grasping a hot coal with the intent of throwing it at someone else; but you are the one who gets burned." When we hold on to anger, it spreads even wider, causing depression, self-doubt, and even more anger. Here are some things you can do that may help you cope with your anger:

- Admit your anger and discover what is prompting it. Take a mental snapshot of the moment. Step back and take the same picture with a panoramic lens. What else is in the picture?

- Can you capture or identify why you feel angry?

- When you think about the aspects of your condition that make you angry, what does your body do in response to the angry thoughts? (for example, breath holding, increased muscle tension, increased blood pressure)

- What are the advantages to you of staying angry? What might be the disadvantages?

- Can you identify ways to suffer less physically because of your anger? (for example, relaxation techniques, breathing through tension while thinking of your anger)

- Can you identify ways to suffer less emotionally because of your anger? (for example, meditation; looking to the future for what you can do, not to the past for what you have lost)

- Write down how you have benefited from the experience of diabetes and how your life is better as a result of what happened. Do not withhold anything, and be as honest as possible.

- Consider the advantages of "benefit-finding." Ask yourself the following (Wiseman, 2009): Does the thing that makes you angry help you:

  - grow stronger or become aware of personal strengths that you didn't realize you had?

  - appreciate certain aspects of your life more than before?

  - become a wiser person?

  - enhance important relationships or end bad ones?

  - become more skilled at communicating your feelings?

  - bolster your confidence?

  - develop into a more compassionate or forgiving person?

  - identify any of your own shortcomings that may stand in the way of your happiness?

- Would it be worth it to communicate your anger calmly and assertively?

- Would it be worth it to modify your expectations?

- Can you develop a more positive attitude and more positive self-talk?

- Can you channel your anger through new activities (exercise, writing, music, painting)?

- One of the most powerful antidotes to anger is forgiveness. If you are angry at yourself, what would it take to forgive yourself? If you are angry at someone else, what would it take to forgive that person?

- Another powerful antidote to anger is empathy. If you are angry at someone else, can you suspend judgment about that person until you have taken the time necessary to gather information, walk in the other person's shoes, and develop a full understanding of his or her viewpoint?

Coping With Anxiety

The hallmark symptom of anxiety is worry. People who suffer from anxiety tend to worry about everything—what their blood sugar readings will be, what will happen at the next doctor's visit, what other people will think of them if they test their blood sugar in public, and what will happen to their health over time. Other symptoms of anxiety include restlessness, muscle tension, irritability, edginess, sleep disturbance, and feeling easily overwhelmed.

The problem with anxiety is that it inhibits our ability to cope with illness. It fosters feelings of powerlessness and lack of control. Worst of all, it disrupts our problem-solving ability. It makes it very difficult for us to engage in flexible, constructive thought when we are faced with a health management obstacle or challenge. Here are some things you can do that may help you cope with your anxiety:

- Talk with a health care provider about the possibility of getting treatment through psychotherapy, medications, or both.

- Reconnect with your body. Feel your feet against the floor. Let your shoulders and neck drop. Observe how it feels not to resist the pull of gravity.

- Engage in relaxation techniques such as listening to a mindfulness meditation CD, practicing deep breathing, or practicing a body scan technique.

- Identify, label, and talk about the anxiety.

- Identify coping resources that you can draw upon when needed.

- Exercise. Just as with depression, research findings have shown that moderate physical activity can be just as effective as medications in helping some people manage mild anxiety symptoms.

- Seek support from others.

- Practice problem solving techniques.

Coping With Fear

While anxiety is often a free-floating collection of worries, fear has a specific target. People with diabetes sometimes fear puncturing their skin with a lancet to get a blood sample for a blood sugar reading. Or they may fear giving their blood sugar meter to their health care provider so the provider can examine the record of recent blood sugar readings. Or they may fear the experience of a low blood sugar level.

The problem with fear is that it leads to avoidance behaviors. Then, when you avoid a certain situation or activity, you cannot receive any information that disconfirms your reason for fear. So, the avoidance intensifies, and your life becomes progressively more limited. The key here is to learn how to "approach, not avoid." Deep breathing or relaxation strategies often help people approach a feared situation with greater comfort. A mental health professional or medical provider can help you create coping thoughts to counteract your specific fear. When you repeatedly approach the feared situation, you will find that the level of fear diminishes over time.

Coping With Guilt

Guilt is an emotion that feels all too familiar to many people with diabetes. There can be many layers of guilt—from guilt due to your sense that it's your fault that you got this disease in the first place, to guilt for all of the diet and exercise rules you have broken, to guilt over each blood sugar rating that is not in the target range. The problem with guilt is that like depression, it can be paralyzing, demoralizing, and exhausting. You are going to need all of your energy to take good care of your health, so consider the following ideas for coping with guilt:

- Guilt is often considered to be a "useless emotion" in that it serves no identifiable purpose. Ask yourself these questions: Is my guilt serving me in any positive way? Is there any aspect of my guilt that I need to keep? If not, can I shift my attention to a more helpful emotion?

- Many times, when we try to push away a feeling like guilt, it only becomes stronger. Instead of trying to "get rid of" guilt, see if you can recognize the feeling when it emerges, allow it to be there, observe it with an attitude of curiosity ("Oh, there it is again—I recognize that feeling!"), AND do what you need to do to manage your health. Having your feelings and taking good care of yourself are NOT incompatible.

- Some individuals worry that if they don't pay enough attention to their guilt, they will somehow slip into "bad behavior" and neglect their diabetes care altogether. If this describes you, imagine how much more energy and motivation you would have if you were motivated by positive emotions (such as hope and optimism) rather than beating yourself up each time you feel like you did something wrong. Shifting to positive motivators might make a dramatic difference to your energy supply.

Homework

Over the next week, notice if depression, anger, anxiety, fear, or guilt come up when you think about your diabetes. If they emerge, see if you can use some of the strategies from this lesson to cope with the emotions.

Lesson Eleven: Manage Frustration, Discouragement, and Hopelessness

"Every great work, every great accomplishment, has been brought into manifestation through holding to the vision, and often just before the big achievement comes apparent failure and discouragement."

-Florence Scovel Shinn

———

Perhaps even more common than emotions like depression and anger are feelings such as frustration, discouragement, defeatism, and hopelessness. In this lesson, you will discover the thinking errors that give rise to these feelings and how to challenge them by generating more helpful thoughts.

Thinking Errors

Many times when we feel frustrated, discouraged, or hopeless, it is because we are making certain "thinking errors" in our mind. Here are some examples of thinking errors that occur in the context of diabetes:

- All-or-nothing thinking (Either I am perfectly healthy, or my whole body is falling apart.)

- Overgeneralization (I always get worse when I try to follow medical advice.)

- Magnification (The tingling in my foot means that I will soon need my foot amputated.)

- Should-statements (I should be able to resist junk food after a long, stressful day at work.)

Why do we develop thinking errors?

- Previous life experiences with illness

- Witnessing the illness experiences of family members or friends

- Cultural beliefs or media messages

- Actual or perceived messages from health care providers

Here are some questions to ask yourself to help identify thinking errors:

What goes through my mind when I think of myself having a chronic illness?

What do I find myself thinking when my health is worse than expected, despite having followed my treatment plan closely?

What thoughts have led me to discontinue my efforts at taking care of my diabetes in the past?

What do I think when despite having followed medical advice, my condition does not improve?

Do I have any concerns, worries, or fears that come to mind when I think about managing my diabetes?

Now, once you've identified the thinking errors, what do you do? Draw a line down the middle of a piece of paper. In the left column, write down the thinking errors. In the right column, see if you can generate some "replacement thoughts" or more balanced, alternative thoughts that help you think about the situation in a more reasonable, constructive way.

Example:

Thinking error

This is unfair. (Magnification?)

Replacement thoughts

Other people have other medical conditions that are just as unfair or even worse.

Dwelling on the unfairness does not help me be any more enthusiastic about my health management.

I could be grateful that scientists know so much more about diabetes today compared to 20 or 30 years ago.

I don't have to be happy about having the condition, nor do I have to believe that it is fair. I can recognize the unfairness and still do what I need to do to take care of myself.

Homework

Choose one thinking error that interferes with your health management, and generate as many replacement thoughts as you can.

Lesson Twelve: Deal With Disappointing Blood Sugar Readings

"The size of your success is measured by the strength of your desire; the size of your dream; and how you handle disappointment along the way."

-Robert Kiyosaki

"We must accept finite disappointment, but never lose infinite hope."

-Martin Luther King, Jr.

―――――――

I have met many individuals with diabetes who told me that they stopped checking their blood sugar readings because they cannot handle the disappointment that accompanies a high reading. In this lesson, you will learn a process that may help you get "unhooked" from thoughts and feelings of self-disappointment.

Challenging Your Thoughts

In order to challenge your thoughts about disappointment, you need to examine them and test them against objective evidence to determine how valid or accurate they are. The process is called cognitive reframing or cognitive restructuring. It involves asking yourself a series of questions to explore whether the thoughts are supported by the available evidence. If they are not (and many of our negative thoughts are not), you generate a more helpful alternative thought. Here are the questions to ask yourself:

- What is actually true about this situation?

- What is the evidence that my thought is true and correct?

- What facts am I forgetting or ignoring?

- What errors am I making in my thinking? (see previous lesson)

- What are the true facts of the situation, and what am I making up or exaggerating?

- What are some other ways to think about this situation?

- If my best friend were having this thought, what would I say to support her?

- If my best friend knew that I was having this thought, what would she say to support me?

- Is there a more positive way to look at this situation?

- Is there any benefit I can find in this situation?

- What practical things could I do to deal with this situation?

- Is the situation really as bad as I am making it out to be?

- What is the worst thing that could happen?

- How likely is it that the worst thing will happen?

- If the worst thing happens, how would I handle it?

- What is probably, most likely, going to happen?

Example:

Original thought

A 280 blood sugar! I just can't get it right.

Alternative thoughts

280 is higher than I would like it to be. But it is just temporary, and I can view it as a learning opportunity. I can go take a walk to improve my reading. A problem-solving approach is going to help me in this moment much more than guilt.

Lesson Thirteen: Manage Setbacks

"In the middle of a difficulty lies opportunity."

-Albert Einstein

"It may sound strange, but many champions are made champions by setbacks."

-Bob Richards

"It isn't the mountain ahead that wears you out; it's the grain of sand in your shoe."

-Robert Service

It is so common for us to feel that we have "failed" when normal obstacles and challenges arise on the path to change. In this lesson, you will consider alternative ways to manage setbacks without getting bogged down in feelings of failure (which can be like a grain of sand in your shoe!). After all, feelings of failure just lead to diminished energy, focus, and motivation, and you're going to need those resources for the journey ahead.

Thinking About Failure Differently

When friends embark on a new endeavor, we bid them "Godspeed," "Good luck," or "Best wishes for success." If we trust the research on personal change, however, it might make more sense to wish them "Good failure."

Failure, it seems, is a necessary part of the change process. As you learned earlier in this book, researchers Prochaska, Norcross, and

DiClemente have demonstrated that people often need to cycle through the stages of the change journey multiple times before they are able to make a change stick (1994). Similarly, psychology professor Richard Wiseman has shown that 88% of all New Year's resolutions end in failure, but many people achieve success after they work on the same resolution for several years in a row (2009).

Chances are, if you are working on a goal that is challenging but desirable, you will encounter hardship somewhere along the way. Chip and Dan Heath describe a tool that can help us adopt reasonable expectations (2010). It's called the "Project Mood Chart," and it was developed by Tim Brown, the CEO at IDEO, which is one of the world's most successful product design firms.

The Project Mood Chart is a U-shaped curve. The peak at the beginning is called "hope," and it represents all of the positive feelings we have at the beginning of a change journey, when we feel inspired, energetic, and ready to take on a challenge. (Think about all of the people whom you've never seen at your gym before but who suddenly show up during the first week of January.)

The peak at the end of the curve is called "confidence," and it represents the sense of achievement and personal efficacy we feel when we have successfully reached our goal.

The valley between the two peaks is filled with negative emotions such as depression, doubt, hopelessness, helplessness, frustration, angst, and feelings of failure. Tim Brown labels this valley "insight."

The main message of the Project Mood Chart is that failure is a natural and essential part of the change process. You cannot trust the energetic charge you feel at the beginning of a project, because what follows is the negative emotional valley. But *the negative emotional valley is what gives us essential insight.* And reminding ourselves that we are building essential insights can help minimize feelings of hopelessness and discouragement.

Remember Carol Dweck's research on "mindset" that we covered in lesson one? Dr. Dweck, who writes about the mindset that helps us achieve great things, tells us that *falling down is learning rather than failing.* And we all know you have to fall down a few times before you can learn to run.

Reflection Questions: What do I say to myself when I fall down? If I am a person who beats myself up mentally each time I fall down, how helpful has that been? Is it worth holding onto that strategy? Or is there a way to view "falling down" as a sign of learning, not failing?

Lapse Versus Relapse

When you are working toward your health-related goal and you experience a setback, it is important to be honest with yourself and evaluate whether the setback signals a lapse or a relapse. A lapse is a temporary detour off the path to change. For example, the day you fail to go out for your regular walk after several days of consistent walking, you've had a lapse. A lapse is a time-limited exception to your normal healthy behavior.

A relapse, on the other hand, is an *ongoing pattern of lapses.* It's not just a temporary detour off the path to change; it's traveling down a different road altogether. For example, when you abandon your daily walks and you're not even trying to get back on track, you've had a relapse. The hopelessness and discouragement that accompany relapse may make it difficult for you to even imagine that you can resume goal-consistent behaviors.

The reason it is important to distinguish between a lapse and a relapse is because they each require a different response. When you have a lapse, you can learn about the obstacle that diverted you off the path, shore up your resources, and return to your action plan. When you have a relapse, however, you will need to reassess your stage of change (see lesson two), because you are likely revisiting an earlier stage of change. Once you determine your current stage of change, you will know what mental tasks will help you move forward again.

The Need for Self-Compassion

There is a lot of psychological research highlighting the importance of self-esteem when dealing with challenges or when working toward goals. Recently, however, there has been evidence that *compassion toward the self* may be even more important than self-esteem when we are facing setbacks.

What does a self-compassionate stance look like when you feel discouraged or hopeless with regard to your diabetes goals? If you fight against your negative feelings, you may get trapped in self-criticism, depression, anxiety, or rumination. However, if you respond to your negative feelings with kindness and understanding, you are able to hold on to your personal initiative and coping efforts, and change flows more naturally.

We'll take a closer look at self-compassion in lesson sixteen. For now, consider this reflection question:

Reflection Question: What would it look like for me to respond to my setbacks with kindness and understanding?

Lesson Fourteen: Increase Acceptance

"It's the awareness…of how you are stuck, that makes you recover."

-Fritz Perls

"We cannot change anything until we accept it. Condemnation does not liberate, it oppresses."

-C. G. Jung

Changing reality requires first accepting the facts of the situation that you are in. Acceptance does not mean resigning yourself to your condition; rather, it means an active embracing of your condition, your starting point, and your emotions so that you can free yourself up to move forward. In this lesson, you will learn ways to increase acceptance, which is a crucial ingredient in the change process.

Reality Acceptance

Are there any aspects of your medical condition that are difficult for you to accept? Perhaps it is difficult to accept that you even have diabetes in the first place. Or, it is difficult to accept that you have not been doing everything you can to manage your health. Many people find it difficult to accept the emotions that accompany diabetes, such as anger, fear, or feelings of loss.

What is the advantage of being able to accept the reality of your situation? First, we know that rejecting and denying reality does not *change* reality. They simply keep you stuck. Second, we know that when you push away reality, you add a layer of suffering on top of your symptoms. The more you fight the aspects of your illness that cannot be changed, the more of your life they take away.

What does reality acceptance involve? Acceptance involves:

- Acknowledging what IS (not what should be)

- Tolerating one moment at a time

- Doing the best you can do, given the reality of the situation (as opposed to trying to control the situation)

- Making an active choice to accept the aspects of your illness that cannot be changed

Acceptance is NOT giving up, passively resigning, or taking a defeatist stance. It does not mean that you are happy about having diabetes. It does not mean that you enjoy having diabetes. It does not mean that you have given up hope of feeling better. It simply means coming to terms with reality so that you can live the vital, engaged, meaningful life you want to live WITH your diabetes.

Consider these tips for increasing your level of acceptance. They are adapted from Diana Lund, survivor of brain injury and author of the book *Remind Me Why I'm Here* (2006):

- Understanding your illness or disability must precede acceptance. Learn as much as you can about your condition.

- Be open-minded. Consider that you are "the same, but different," and persist in learning as much as you can about how you have changed.

- Allow yourself to feel anger, sadness, frustration, or other negative emotions.

- Allow yourself to walk through your grief, not around it.

- Get support from your family, friends, medical team, and/or support group.

- Take a self-growth perspective. Remember that coping with illness is a process or a "work-in-progress."

- Make a list of what you've lost forever, what you've gained, and what you can work on.

- Spend some time imagining what it would look like when you've achieved an increase in self-acceptance. What would be different inside yourself? How would you think differently about things? Feel differently about things?

- See yourself as courageous and adaptable. Believe that if you nurture these qualities, they will see you through the difficult times.

Reflection Question: What would it mean for me to learn how to live my life with diabetes, rather than letting it take my life away from me?

Homework

Answer the following questions:

If you were to come to greater acceptance of the things you do NOT have control over, how would your situation change?

Would it free up some of your energy? What would you use that energy for?

Think about the goal you are working on as you read through this book. How might non-acceptance be negatively impacting your ability to address this goal?

Lesson Fifteen: Challenge Excuses

"An excuse is worse and more terrible than a lie...."

-Alexander Pope

"We lie to ourselves, in order that we may still have the excuse of ignorance, the alibi of stupidity and incomprehension, possessing which we can continue with a good conscience to commit and tolerate the most monstrous crimes."

-Aldous Huxley

———⊱※———

Human beings can be masters of the art of excuses, allowing self-defeating thinking habits to interfere with their best efforts at personal change. In this lesson, you will identify the most common excuses that interfere with your efforts to take care of your physical health. Then, you will learn the steps you can take to transform self-defeating habits into goal-congruent thinking habits.

Common Excuses

Dr. Wayne Dyer, a psychologist, author, teacher, and speaker famous for his presentations on public television, has created a catalog of the excuses that people use most often (2009). Although there are many, many different excuses, they all boil down to about eighteen fundamental categories. Let's look at the ones that are used most commonly when your health management efforts aren't going the way you want them to:

- It is too difficult.

- It will take too long.

- It's not my nature.

- I'm too old for this.

- I'm not strong enough.

- It's too big of a problem.

- I don't have the energy.

- I'm too busy.

- It's my personal family history (or "It's in my genes").

Reflection Question: What excuse(s) do you use to avoid taking good care of your health?

Challenging Excuses

What is one area of your diabetes management in which you need to be more honest with yourself? Now, consider this: What if, for all intents and purposes your excuses cease to exist and there is no possible way you can fall back on them anymore? What would your life look like without these excuses? Without these excuses, how would you feel? How would your thoughts be different? How would your behaviors be different?

Another question to ask yourself is this: "What are the things I am saying to myself that are allowing my unhealthy behaviors to continue?" This question allows you to identify how your excuses become "facilitating statements" that make your bad habits seem reasonable (and therefore acceptable). These facilitating thoughts are a setup for failure, because they allow your bad habits to continue unchecked.

It can be helpful to make a list of your facilitating thoughts, and then for each one, challenge yourself to develop a more helpful response.

Example:

Facilitating thought

I deserve to treat myself.

Helpful response

I do deserve to treat myself, but I have a problem of sticking to my diet and keeping my blood sugars in a healthy range. So in the long run, the nicest thing I can do for myself is to care for my health and reward myself with fun activities, not food. Once I am engaged in a fun activity, I won't be thinking about my temptation to eat something that I shouldn't eat.

Homework

Choose one facilitating thought that sabotages your health management, and generate as many helpful responses as you can.

Lesson Sixteen: Treat Yourself With Compassion

"Lack of forgiveness causes almost all of our self-sabotaging behavior."

-Mark Victor Hansen

———⟨≋⟩———

It has been well-established that self esteem is important when you are dealing with challenges or working toward personal goals. Recently, however, there has been evidence that *compassion toward the self* may be even more important than self esteem when you are facing hard times. In this lesson, you will learn more about the pathways to greater self-compassion.

What Is Self-Compassion?

It seems like it is human nature to fight against difficult emotions, to push them away, and to tuck them into the back corners of the mind. Unfortunately, though, the more you fight emotional pain, the more you tend to get trapped in it. An entirely different approach is to allow emotional pain to be present and to treat yourself with kindness and understanding at these times, just as you would treat a dear friend who is suffering.

If you can't generate a good-enough reason to treat yourself with compassion, perhaps the research on the topic will convince you. It has been demonstrated that people who have more self-compassion are less depressed, anxious, self-critical, and perfectionistic. They enjoy many benefits in their lives compared to their non-self-compassionate counterparts. These benefits include more happiness, wisdom, personal initiative, optimism, life satisfaction, and social connectedness.

Pathways to Self-Compassion

Here are some ideas for cultivating self-compassion. These ideas come from Christopher Germer's book, *The Mindful Path to Self-Compassion: Freeing Yourself From Destructive Thoughts and Emotions* (2009).

- Physical pathways

  - Soften the breath, perhaps through mindful breathing exercises.

  - Soften the muscles and tissues of the body, perhaps through relaxation techniques.

  - Participate in good physical self-care.

- Mental pathways

  - Allow your thoughts to come and go more freely.

  - Use a visual image to create mental space (e.g., imagining your thoughts as leaves flowing down a stream).

  - Put things in perspective (e.g., asking yourself what you value most in life).

- Emotional pathways

  - Increase acceptance of painful emotions instead of fighting against them.

  - Take the perspective of others to learn how to forgive yourself (e.g., "What would my best friend say?").

  - Treat yourself to enjoyable activities.

- Relational pathways

    - Connect with others.

    - Reduce the suffering of others whenever you can.

    - Forgive yourself for how you have harmed others.

- Spiritual pathways

    - Take the time to cultivate your faith or your spiritual values.

    - Connect with the miracle of everyday life, accepting and embracing the imperfections that you notice.

<u>Homework</u>

Answer the following questions:

How do you care for yourself physically?

Can you think of new ways to release the tension and stress that builds up in your body?

How do you care for your mind, especially when you're under stress?

Is there a new strategy you'd like to try to let your thoughts come and go more easily?

How do you already care for yourself emotionally?

Is there something new you'd like to try?

How or when do you relate to others that brings you genuine happiness?

Is there any way that you'd like to enrich these connections?

What do you do to care for yourself spiritually?

If you've been neglecting your spiritual side, is there anything you'd like to remember to do?

Lesson Seventeen: Arrange Social Support

"Here is the basic rule for winning success. Let's mark it in the mind and remember it. The rule is: Success depends on the support of other people. The only hurdle between you and what you want to be is the support of other people."

-David Joseph Schwartz

There is abundant evidence that social support is crucial in helping us get through difficult times. In this lesson, you learn how to ask others for the specific kind of support that you need from them as you work toward your health-management goals.

Coaching Others

Some of the most interesting and lively discussions we have in my diabetes group center around the issue of living with diabetes in the context of relationships: with family members, friends, coworkers, neighbors, and acquaintances. You don't live with your diabetes alone; you live with it in a social context. Sometimes, members of your social network hold strong opinions, inaccurate beliefs, or judgments about diabetes, and they aren't afraid to voice their thoughts. Other times, members of your social network truly connect with your experience and offer much-needed support and understanding.

Given the wide variety of reactions and responses other people have to your medical condition, it is helpful for you to identify what kind of responses are most helpful to you, and *what specific type of support you prefer.* How do you want your spouse or partner to support you? For example, do you want him or her to give you verbal reminders to check your blood sugar at meal times? If so, what *exactly* should he or she say? Or do you prefer that he or she not say anything at all, because any prompt would make you feel nagged or harassed?

How do you handle the meal-planning in your household? The grocery shopping? Are there any rules about which snack foods are allowed in your house? Are there any specific supportive statements you would want to hear from your friends or coworkers? How do you handle the issue of treats that coworkers bring into the workplace to celebrate special occasions? How do you manage your diabetes when you go out to eat with your friends? Are there any specific discussions you need to have about these topics? What do you want to ask for?

Think of yourself as "coaching" others about the things that are most helpful to you. Many people want to be helpful and supportive, but they simply don't know how. Or they are afraid that they will offend you if they ask about your health. As the person with diabetes, you can be proactive and positive about these issues, and you can initiate open, problem-solving conversations with your friends and family.

Reflection Question: Consider that the type of support you need will **change** *as you progress through the stages of change. What type of support will you need in the contemplation versus the preparation versus the action stage?*

Choosing Your Support People

The other day, one of my patients took a crumpled piece of paper out of her wallet and told me that on the paper, I had written a question for her to ask herself on a regular basis. She said the question became a very important part of her daily self-reflection. The question was simple: "What kind of people do you want around you?" She said she started to realize that every day we have a choice.

We can surround ourselves with people who are negative, critical, and cynical of our change efforts, or we can find people who are positive, encouraging, and supportive—people who truly believe in us. When it comes to your diabetes management, it is well worth it to identify the important people in your life who fall in the latter category.

Reflection Questions: Who believes in your ability to improve your self care and health management and will support and encourage you no matter what? How can you make sure you have regular contact with these people?

Homework

Answer the following questions:

How have my relationships with my spouse/partner, children, friends, coworkers, and family members changed on account of my diabetes?

How can I "coach" others about my diabetes, my needs, and my capabilities? How can I be sure that my friendships are not dominated by talk about my illness? How can I be sure that I am still being a good friend to others?

How can I improve my communication with the significant people in my life? How can I demonstrate that I am trying to understand their side of things? How can I put myself in their shoes and understand that they are affected by my diabetes, too?

Who is one person who can support my change journey, and what specific kind of help do I want from him or her?

Lesson Eighteen: Be Resilient

"You're alive. Do something. The directive in life, the moral imperative was so uncomplicated. It could be expressed in single words, not complete sentences. It sounded like this: Look. Listen. Choose. Act."

-Barbara Hall

———✦———

In this lesson, you will learn about the characteristics of resilient individuals and people who actively cope with a difficult situation or health challenge. You will learn how to bring these strategies for resilience into your own change process.

What Is Resilience?

Researchers have spent the last two or three decades studying individuals who do well in life despite the fact that they lived through some kind of adversity, trauma, risk, or difficult event. They label these individuals as "resilient" and seek to understand what makes them unique.

Many individuals who deal with illness or disability may be labeled as resilient, as well (see Bonanno, 2004; Elliott, Kurylo, & Rivera, 2002; Tugade & Fredrickson, 2004). Famous examples include Helen Keller, Lance Armstrong, and Christopher Reeve. Here are some factors that predict who will be resilient and who will not when dealing with an illness or medical condition:

- *Earlier behavior*: People who took good care of their physical and emotional health before they developed a chronic illness will be more likely to take good care of themselves after the onset of illness.

- *Social support*: People who have a good support network and fill their lives with friends who can provide both informational and emotional support are more resilient in dealing with illness.

- *Locus of control*: People who have an internal locus of control (meaning that they believe they are responsible for the outcomes in their lives) are more resilient than people who have an external locus of control (meaning that they believe that outside forces such as fate or luck determine their destiny).

- *Problem-solving orientation*: Individuals who approach the challenges of illness with a problem-solving stance are more resilient than their counterparts who lack this skill.

- *Hope*: People who are hopeful identify and pursue meaningful goals even in times of distress. This gives them a greater sense of control and leads to better coping and resilience.

- *Goal orientation*: Individuals who actively set and pursue goals remain more resilient in the face of a challenge such as illness or disability.

- *Positive emotion-inducing coping*: When a person is skilled in positive emotion-inducing coping, he or she is able to find positive meaning in negative circumstances and able to create positive emotions to bounce back from a hardship or setback. It is easy to see how this makes a person more resilient in coping with illness.

- *Hardiness*: People who are labeled as "hardy" tend to see problems as challenges rather than obstacles. They remain committed to their values and goals, and they perceive a sense of control over the outcome of their efforts.

Homework

Answer the following questions:

Who is a person who demonstrates some of the qualities of resilience described in this lesson? How can I be more like this person?

What ultimately gets me through the tough times in dealing with my diabetes?

What would it mean for me to make the choice to be resilient?

What one thing can I change right now in my life to improve my chances of "bouncing back" after a setback?

Lesson Nineteen: Be an Optimalist

"The greatest mistake a man can make is to be afraid of making one."

-Elbert Hubbard

"Failure is an inescapable part of life and a critically important part of any successful life. We learn to walk by falling, to talk by babbling, to shoot a basket by missing, and to color the inside of a square by scribbling outside the box. Those who intensely fear failing end up falling short of their potential. We either learn to fail or we fail to learn."

-Tal Ben-Shahar

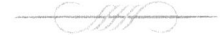

In this lesson, you will learn how to guard against perfectionism when it interferes with your change efforts.

Perfectionism Versus Optimalism

Psychologist Tal Ben-Shahar makes a distinction between a perfectionist and an "optimalist" in his book, *The Pursuit of Perfect* (2009):

The Perfectionist	The Optimalist
Change as a straight line	Change as an irregular spiral
Fear of failure	Failure as feedback
All-or-nothing thinking	Nuanced, complex thinking
Defensive	Open to suggestions
Fault-finder	Benefit-finder
Harsh toward self and others	Forgives self & others
Rigid, static	Adaptable, dynamic

Ben-Shahar writes that the more qualities of perfectionism you exhibit, the more vulnerable you are to problems such as depression, anxiety, and low self-esteem. On the other hand, the more qualities of optimalism you exhibit, the better able you are to learn, grow, and ultimately do well in the change process. You may even enjoy the journey of change, because you are not overcome by procrastination, paralysis, and diminished motivation and desire.

Imagine what this means for your diabetes management. When you are defensive, unforgiving toward yourself, and rigid in your thinking (for example, "I need to do this 100% correctly or it's not worth doing at all), how much initiative and enthusiasm do you have for your diabetes care? How does that compare to the times when you are flexible, open, and ready to take the detours of the change journey in stride?

Homework

Answer the following questions:

When does perfectionism show up in my diabetes management efforts?

What do I gain from being a perfectionist at these times?

What price do I pay for being a perfectionist at these times?

Which aspects of perfectionism do I want to keep?

Which elements of perfectionism do I want to get rid of?

Lesson Twenty: Prevent Relapse

"A stitch in time saves nine."

"It wasn't raining when Noah built the ark."

"Even if you're on the right track, you'll get run over if you just sit there."

Just when you think you've succeeded at making an important life change, circumstances will arise that challenge your commitment and confidence. In this final lesson, you will learn to identify the signals or clues that you are regressing in your change efforts, and you will design a relapse prevention plan to help you get back on track.

What Is Relapse Prevention?

You are now prepared to design a plan for preventing or coping with future diabetes-related problems. The term for that is "relapse prevention." It is the task of thinking ahead during your good periods about how you might handle the more difficult times. We engage in relapse prevention because there is the potential that when certain stressful situations come along in the future, they may lead you to abandon your newly-acquired positive habits.

Building an Individualized Relapse Prevention Plan

Think back over the book. What did you learn that was most meaningful to you? What were you able to put into practice and benefit from? How did you change? How did your efforts lead to change?

What might get in the way of your efforts to continue with the skills you have learned in the book?

- Noncompliance/nonadherence

- Faulty memory

- Lack of motivation

- Failure to be supported by the environment

- Additional health problems

- Getting discouraged that "nothing works"

- Feelings that "it should be better/easier by now"

- Lack of encouragement from those around you

- Increased personal stress

- Increased pain

- Increased fatigue

- Time constraints

- Inconvenience

- Distraction

- Other:

What high-risk situations are coming up in your life that might undermine your efforts at good diabetes self-care?

- Life transitions

- Illnesses, accidents, surgery

- Special environments (workplaces, living environments, etc.)

- Travel

- Social occasions

- Stressful events

- Other:

For each high-risk situation you identified, consider how you could get yourself back on track.

Problem:

Solution:

Problem:

Solution:

Problem:

Solution:

What is your panic plan? Instead of panicking when your diabetes self-care efforts fail, you can refer to a detailed list of things you have identified to be helpful for the mind, body, and spirit. Making this list ahead of time will help you take action when things go off-course. The more specific you make the plan, the easier it will be to follow. Make a list of the resources, skills, and techniques you have.

Panic plan for my mind...

Panic plan for my body...

Panic plan for my spirit...

What are your healthy pleasures? Chronic illness can cause us to eliminate the fun from life. This is a serious mistake; we all need a daily dose of pleasure. Stay open to enjoyment. Keep a long list of things you like to do, and refer to it whenever you start feeling overwhelmed by your diabetes.

My healthy pleasures are:

What will you do when you have a bad day and cannot seem to get back on track with your diabetes self-care efforts, no matter what you do? Be careful how you are thinking about, judging, or labeling yourself or your efforts. Remember that we all have setbacks. Change is a winding road. Tomorrow will probably be better. Your path to improvement may follow an up-and-down course. Remember the "big picture," as well as the upward spiral of change.

What I will do *when I have a bad day and cannot seem to get back on track with diabetes self-care efforts:*

Coping thoughts I will think *when I have a bad day and cannot seem to get back on track with diabetes self-care efforts:*

Not all possible problematic circumstances can be anticipated. Rather, the goal is for you to increase your confidence that you have what it takes to respond appropriately to problems. Write yourself an encouraging statement about your ability to cope with challenges.

An encouraging statement about my confidence in the ability to cope with challenges:

Minor setbacks are inevitable and do not signal total failure. Watch out for hopeless thinking or all-or-nothing thinking (for example, "Well, my diabetes is not responding to my efforts to manage it, so I might as well give up on my active coping efforts.")

How to remind myself that minor setbacks do not mean total failure:

Don't forget to enlist the assistance of significant others.

Who are the supportive people in my life to whom I can make myself accountable for further practice of my new skills?

How can I keep the change going now that I have finished this book?

Best wishes for your continued change efforts! I would love to hear about your progress. You can contact me through my website at www.heidibeckman.com.

References and Additional Readings

Bandura, A. (1997). <u>Self-efficacy: The exercise of control</u>. New York: W. H. Freeman and Company.

Baumeister, R. F., Bratslavsky, E., Muraven, M., & Tice, D. M. (1998). Ego depletion: Is the active self a limited resource? <u>Journal of Personality and Social Psychology, 74,</u> 1252-1265.

Ben-Shahar, T. (2009). <u>The pursuit of perfect: How to stop chasing perfection and start living a richer, happier life</u>. New York: McGraw Hill.

Bonanno, G. A. (2004). Loss, trauma, and human resilience: Have we underestimated the capacity to thrive after extremely aversive events? <u>American Psychologist, 59,</u> 20-28.

Bridle, C., Riemsma, R. P., Pattenden, J., Sowden, A. J., Mather, L., Watt, I. S., & Walker, A. (2005). Systematic review of the effectiveness of health behavior interventions based on the transtheoretical model. <u>Psychology and Health, 20,</u> 283-301.

Canning, I., Sherman, E., & Unwin, G. (Producers), & Hooper, T. (Director). (2010). The king's speech [Motion Picture]. United Kingdom: Seesaw Films.

Dahl, J. & Lundgren, T. (2006). <u>Living beyond your pain: Using acceptance and commitment therapy to ease chronic pain</u>. Oakland, CA: New Harbinger.

Duckworth, A. L., Peterson, C., Matthews, M. D., & Kelly, D. R. (2007). Grit: Perseverance and passion for long-term goals. <u>Journal of Personality and Social Psychology, 92,</u> 1087-1101.

Dweck, C. (2006). Mindset: The new psychology of success. New York: Ballantine.

Dyer, W. W. (2009). Excuses begone: How to change lifelong, self-defeating thinking habits. Carlsbad, California: Hay House, Inc.

Elliott, T. R., Kurylo, M., & Rivera, P. (2002). Positive growth following acquired physical disability. In C. R. Snyder & S. J. Lopez (Eds.), Handbook of Positive Psychology (pp. 687-699). New York: Oxford University Press.

Germer, C. K. (2009). The mindful path to self-compassion: Freeing yourself from destructive thoughts and emotions. New York: Guilford.

Grandey, A. A. (2000). Emotional regulation in the workplace: A new way to conceptualize emotional labor. Journal of Occupational Health Psychology, 5, 95-110.

Haidt, J. (2006). The happiness hypothesis: Finding modern truth in ancient wisdom. New York: Basic Books.

Heath, C., & Heath, D. (2010). Switch: How to change things when change is hard. New York: Broadway Books.

Hollenbeck, J., Williams, C., & Klein, H. (1989). An empirical examination of the antecedents of commitment to difficult goals. Journal of Applied Psychology, 74, 18-23.

Houser-Marko, L., & Sheldon, K. (2006). Motivating behavioral persistence: The self-as-doer construct. Personality and Social Psychology Bulletin, 32, 1037-1049.

Locke, E. A. (1996). Motivation through conscious goal setting. Applied and Preventive Psychology, 5, 117-124.

Locke, E. A., & Latham, G. P. (2002). Building a practically useful theory of goal setting and task motivation: A 35-year odyssey. American Psychologist, 57, 705-717.

Lund, D. (2006). Remind me why I'm here: Sifting through sudden loss of memory and judgment. Published by iUniverse, inc.

McGonigal, K. (2011). The willpower instinct: How self-control works, why it matters, and what you can do to get more of it. New York: Avery.

Muraven, M., Tice, D. M., & Baumeister, R. F. (1998). Self-control as a limited resource: Regulatory depletion patterns. Journal of Personality and Social Psychology, 74, 774-789.

Noar, S. M., Benac, C. N., & Harris, M. S. (2007). Does tailoring matter? Meta-analytic review of tailored print health behavior change interventions. Psychological Bulletin, 133, 673-693.

Norcross, J. C., Ratzin, A. C., & Payne, D. (1989). Ringing in the New Year: The change process and reported outcomes of resolutions. Addictive Behaviors, 14, 205-212.

Prochaska, J. O., Norcross, J. C., & DiClemente, C. C. (1994). Changing for good: A revolutionary six-stage program for overcoming bad habits and moving your life positively forward. New York: HarperCollins.

Prochaska, J. O., & Velicer, W. F. (1997). The transtheoretical model of health behavior change. American Journal of Health Promotion, 12, 38-48.

Salmela, S., Poskiparta, M., Kasila, K., Vahasarja, K., & Vanhala, M. (2009). Transtheoretical model-based dietary interventions in primary care: A review of the evidence in diabetes. Health Education Research, 24, 237-252.

Segerstrom, S. C., & Solberg Nes, L. (2007). Heart rate variability indexes self-regulatory strength, effort, and fatigue. Psychological Science, 18, 275-281.

Thaler, R. H., & Sunstein, C. R. (2008). Nudge: Improving decisions about health, wealth, and happiness. New York: Penguin.

Tugade, M. M., & Fredrickson, B. L. (2004). Resilient individuals use positive emotions to bounce back from negative emotional experiences. Journal of Personality and Social Psychology, 86, 320-333.

Vohs, K. D., Baumeister, R. F., Schmeichel, B. J., Twenge, J. M., Nelson, N. M., & Tice, D. M. (2008). Making choices impairs subsequent self-control: A limited-resource account of decision making, self-regulation, and active initiative. Journal of Personality and Social Psychology, 94, 883-898.

Weick, K. (1984). Small wins. American Psychologist, 39, 40-49.

Wiseman, R. (2009). 59 Seconds: Think a little, change a lot. New York: Alfred A. Knopf.

***

www.ingramcontent.com/pod-product-compliance
Lightning Source LLC
Chambersburg PA
CBHW072320290526
45794CB00002B/714